STAYING STRONGER LONGER
with
WONDERFUL
WAYS WITH WEIGHTS

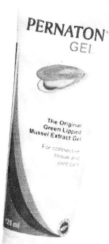
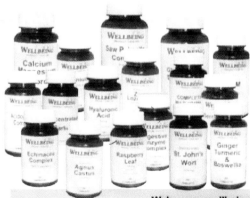

Authors Pauline Eborall
and Patricia Furber

PUBLISHED BY THE KINTBURY
PUBLISHING COMPANY
AND THE SOLE PROPERTY OF THE AUTHORS

A book of easy, illustrated, exercises
and dietary tips to help you stay strong
and avoid some of the hazards of the ageing process.

©
ISBN NO. 0-9554605-2-2

Whilst the author has personally found
the information and exercises contained in this book, a successful regime, it
must be realised that each individual's suitability for exercise and diet may
depend on many differing factors.

It is very important, therefore,
that your medical practitioner should be consulted to decide your suitability
for such a programme. This is particularly important if you are in any of the
following categories:-

Unexercised
Elderly
Taking Medication
Suffering from any Medical Condition
Unsure of your suitability for the Exercises

This book should not be considered or used as an alternative to medical
advice or treatment and the author cannot be held responsible for any actions
taken by a reader as a result of any dependence on the information, including
any errors or omissions, found in the text, diagrams or photographs in this
book, which must be taken entirely at the reader's own risk.

FOREWORD

When I first researched exercise for the over 50's age group, eventually succeeding and then self-publishing Wonderful Ways with Weights in 2006, it was following a long search for exercises that could be commenced at any age and any standard of fitness (or unfitness). Because of my own unsatisfactory experiences as a middle aged woman seeking fitness at gyms and classes, I aimed the exercises towards women - totally ignoring the men in our lives who want and need to attain and retain fitness too. The incidence of men diagnosed with osteoporosis is rising so it is an important issue and one that I have rectified with this updated version.

The exercises discovered and successfully practised for many years apply equally to everyone at any age for in youth exercise is important in building a strong body to last throughout a, hopefully, long life and for the mature person to maintain or regain lost strength. However, even if we have not maintained exercise throughout life, the building blocks remain and can be activated again to build strength, which is what this book is all about.

The exercises are easy to do and can all be done at home, they can be commenced at each individual's current level of fitness, however poor or great that may be, progress is made and strength gained with each exercise session, using the strength gained by the previous session. If you already exercise, add strength exercises to your programme to boost bone and muscle growth.

If you approach the exercise routine sensibly and do not attempt too much too soon, you can gain great new strength in muscles which had forgotten how to work, and also increase bone strength, aided by an adequate proportion of calcium and Vitamin D. The whole body benefits from strength exercise, posture improves, breathing and digestion, circulation and the elimination process improve. Great benefits are found in flexibility and joint mobility.

When first writing the book I did not realise that there were so many older people, all of whom had disappointing experiences in their forays into exercise, very like my own, who were anxious to exercise, but did not know quite what they should be doing. This realisation firstly followed an interview on Woman's Hour and secondly from a feature in Arthritis Today magazine. The immediate public response to both was amazing. Many of the callers had found, like myself, that most gyms and exercise classes did not offer fitness regimes suitable for the unfit, older person and there was not enough readily available guidance on what type of exercise was needed to commence exercising, attempting to slow down the ageing process and help us stay strong as long as possible. What also became apparent at that time was that most of the callers who responded to the radio programme and the magazine article had become so discouraged that they had totally given up on the idea of exercise.

This strengthened my resolve to publish the successful outcome of my research, together with illustrated exercises. I approached several publishing companies, who returned the manuscript for the reason that the age group I was targeting was too small to be commercial and also was not as commercially attractive as exercise books for the young. At this stage I decided to self publish. I did so and the book has been in demand from the over 50's to over 80's, popular with people who are fit and wish to exercise to remain so and with those who already suffer ill health from one or some of the ageing diseases, arthritis being the prime example, but who are able to carry out some degree of exercise (even from a chair) – hence this second edition which I have updated.

I had spent two years researching the type of exercise needed for keeping a strong body and having discovered the strength exercises which did exactly that, practised them for a year with friends, from ages of 40 – 80. We all benefited so much, gradually gaining strength and improving general health that we have all carried on exercising.

Typical findings of research, taken from studies being undertaken throughout the Western world, are that many of the physical failings attributed to ageing and declining health are very often the result of inactivity, which may be reversed by strength exercises and diet.

It has long been believed that ageing brings muscle weakness and it has come to be expected, but research shows that muscle weakness (sarcopenia) which means the deterioration and loss of muscle tissue, experienced by older people with a sedentary lifestyle, who do not undertake strength exercise, is to blame rather than age. Physical activity is vital for everyone but for the 50+ age group cardio vascular exercise alone is not enough. Many over 50's think that walking or swimming are sufficient, but strength exercises are necessary too, to keep all bones and muscles activated and strong. This can make the difference between acceleration of the ageing process and all it's ills, or, opting for strength and lasting good health, enabling one to lead an active, fulfilled and independent life for as long as possible by improving strength, balance and stamina. The risk of obesity, high blood pressure, diabetes, osteoporosis, stroke, depression, colon cancer and premature ageing is greatly reduced by getting physical.

We are fortunate that muscle is amazingly adaptable and even following years of inactivity, it can grow strong again if it is stressed by strength exercises. It is reassuring to know that, if exercise is regular and progressive, strength can be maintained and improved, even by the 80's and 90's age group.

You do not need a gym - you can do it all at home if you wish.

With the advances made by medical science, we should all be living healthier and longer lives, but the former is not happening; this is thought to be mainly due to poor diet and lack of exercise. Both are things that we can do something about and it is important NOT to wait until failing health alerts us that something is going wrong. Muscle weakness and bone frailty are both insidious and are aspects of ageing and inactivity that we should be aware of; they progress slowly 'behind the scenes' and only make themselves known when they have reached an acute state.

It is far more beneficial to be aware and take precautions now, if fitness and good appearance are to be retained and some of the dire consequences of the ageing process avoided. What are YOU doing about it?

You may already exercise and if so, try adding strength exercise to your programme to benefit bone strength. You may find that the very easy, gentle start for beginners advocated in the book is beneath your capabilities, but it is easy to adapt the programme, using heavier weights, more repeats, to suit your own level.

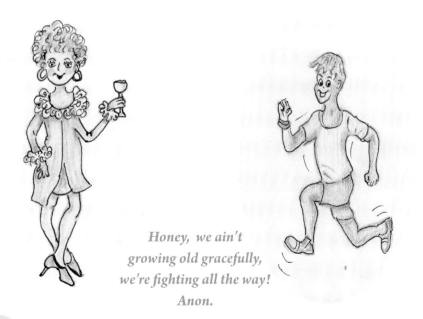

Honey, we ain't growing old gracefully, we're fighting all the way!
Anon.

INTRODUCTION

Older age comes as a surprise to us all; it is one of the things that happen to others, not to us. It is a shock when, having skipped merrily through thirties, forties, fifties and perhaps into sixties too, we actually face the reality that middle age or even old age is lurking around the corner. We realise that we too may become vulnerable to some of the unattractive aspects of ageing, such as joint stiffness, high blood pressure, low bone density, heart problems. This is the time that we begin to take notice of family weaknesses and wonder if we also could become victims.

We read and hear on a daily basis that exercise and a good diet help to fight the ageing process, but just which exercise regime or what class we should join to achieve this can be another story. Sorting out a suitable exercise routine can be difficult, time consuming and discouraging, so much so that it may seem easier to yield to the disadvantages that ageing can bring and do nothing at all.

If you are older and unfit, joining a gym can be daunting, for although an induction course is always insisted upon by the management, this usually consists of a quick tour of the machines and other facilities, with a soon to be forgotten demonstration, followed by the rapid exit of the instructor and you are on your own wondering where to start. Very often there are younger, slimmer, fitter females requiring attention and young male gym instructors are after all only human! This happened to me on my first venture into a gym, I had thought that I had done the difficult part, made the decision to become fit, joined a fitness centre, paid, and had the induction course. However, I felt, rather like Alice, wandering through the looking glass into a strange world, where everyone else in the room knew exactly what they were doing, whilst I stood around wondering what on earth to do with the strange equipment and how I could possibly do it anyway, without causing injury. Also it was rather embarrassing to be the object of curiosity by the much younger, obviously experienced and, rather glamorous Lycra clad exercisers, surrounding me. I made one or two feeble attempts to conquer the tortuous machines, prior to removing myself from the scene, by then determining I had made a mistake and that the obvious thing to do was join a fitness class. I tried several classes, but they tended to be designed for 'across the board fitness' not particularly geared to the older, unfit exerciser; perhaps with some arthritis or joint stiffness and low energy etc, whilst many classmates were at least 20 years younger and bubbling with energy. I found that my energy rapidly expired, often during the 'warm up' period whilst everyone else was skipping around the studio, raring to go on to greater things, I was wondering 'how much longer is this class going to last' and yearning for the floor exercises to begin, when I could lie down and regain my breath. Hopefully the instructor would announce' anyone with back problems please sit this one out' and I could sink gratefully to the floor, ignoring the fact that my back was fine but that I had actually already given my all and had no energy left! Does this sound familiar? Have you been there? I became expert at always taking up a position at the side or rear of the room nearest the door, ready to make a quick exit if the class proved inappropriate. Never, ever to return.

I was several times given programmes, but my experience was that they were far too intensive. I knew that I had to get fit in a gradual manner, before I could 'Keep Fit'.

Then began a search of bookshops for fitness books or videos; again all seemed geared towards the young, already fit individual, which alone was enough to send me zooming past the 'fitness' section to pick up the latest best seller, rush home and collapse on the sofa with a glass of wine, feeling that perhaps I should forget the whole thing.

However, I realised that I must continue the search if I wanted to progress into fitness and reasoned that there must be something out there which would enable me to become fit gradually, without risking life and limb. I began to contact fitness instructors, searching the internet and learning of studies in progress around the western world researching the ageing process and what could be done to counteract it. I was able to follow this research via the Internet and this is how I eventually discovered strength exercise and realised that such exercise is essential if we are to stay as strong as possible through middle age and into a reasonably active old age, and how it can improve existing medical conditions and wellbeing. I devised my programme, which allowed strength in muscles, and renewed bone growth to take place progressively commencing at virtually any level of fitness.

My regime, is gentle, gradual and you never need push yourself beyond your current level of fitness, it is a continuous process, by exercising regularly you are using the strength gained in the previous sessions to progress, in two to three weeks you will notice that you are gaining strength, your energy is increasing and you will want to continue improving. Moreover, it is not competitive; there is no embarrassment that you cannot keep up with the rest of the class, or the person beside you on a treadmill. You will be always be exercising within your own limits, be it at home or at the gym.

WHY EXERCISE?

As 50's progress into 60's, particularly if we have always lead a sedentary life, energy levels can begin to flag, the suppleness that we have always taken for granted starts to disappear, aches and pains become evident, blood pressure can rise, and from an appearance point of view, is it possible that a trim waistline is disappearing into widening hips and a distinctly rounded tummy and an always uplifted bosom may be heading in a southwards direction too? At this time it may also be prudent to opt for fashion styles that not only cover the arms but also flow down over the waistline Perhaps we may find that a waistline measurement for a pair of trousers far exceeds an inside leg measurement.   It is definitely time to take action.

Because we all want to be healthy, active and enjoy a long, productive life, we need to make sure that our feet are not planted on a slippery slope that sedentary living can mean, it can be a route to rapid ageing, when what we need to be doing is pushing back the ageing process, delaying the time when we need to succumb to multiple medication or enforced inactivity. To maximise the bonus of longer life expectancy that medical science now promises, we need to do everything possible to ensure we remain fit enough to enjoy it by staying stronger longer, being active for as long as possible and making the most of those extra years.

Exercise can also actually lift your mental state and alleviate depression. You will find that you cannot worry whilst you are exercising and your psychological strength can increase.

Exercise cannot solve your problems but it can put you in a stronger position mentally to cope with them; very often you can find that you are able to logically and clearly deal with what can have seemed an insurmountable problem.

Life is sweet, horizons have never been wider, there are so many things that we can do if we have the energy and the inclination.

There are some very easy things you can do to help stay strong and healthy throughout your life. It is not a fact that we have to accept muscle loss and weakness and failing bone density, this is more to do with inactivity than age. You can stay active and feel good, look good and stay mobilised through the middle years and well into old age, improving many existing health conditions. With just a little effort you can do the following:-

Reduce:
stress, weight, blood pressure, tension, pain, arthritic pain, cholesterol, impact on joints, risk of injury and medication needs.

Increase:
strength and flexibility,
range of motion and endurance, muscle tone and quality, energy, circulation, balance, coordination, digestion,
self esteem and enjoyment of life.

You can gain a feeling of well-being, improve your sleeping pattern and mentally and physically experience the turnaround of the ageing process.

Personally we have gained undreamt of benefits from strength exercise and we want to share them with you, these are some of those benefits:-

Increased muscle strength and tone
Reduced stress
Improved circulation
Improved posture and balance
Prevention of Osteo-arthritis
and other 'ageing' diseases.
Improved immune system
Lower blood pressure and Lower cholesterol
Depression and anxiety alleviated
Increased joint mobility
Reduction of arthritic pain
Prolonged active life
Looking younger and more shapely – exercise
burns off fat.

As your general health improves you will find other improvements following on. Of prime importance is posture; by improving posture you will not be working against your body by slumping, squeezing and squashing internal organs, for example; imagine the difficult task the lungs have when they have to fight to expand against a round shouldered droop – it's jolly hard work.

Think also of the unfortunate digestive system, trying to digest a meal and being hampered and squeezed out of recognition by poor posture; the kidneys and liver will not be having an easy time either. The energy wasted by maintaining poor posture could be well used elsewhere, allowing you to enjoy the more interesting things in life.

BE KIND TO YOUR BODY –
THERE IS NO DRESS REHEARSAL FOR LIFE

There are many interests and hobbies to be enjoyed. However, we need to be fit enough and have the energy to do so. We all want to live longer, be healthy and feel and look younger. We will show you how to do it in easy stages, it is just a question of fitting a little exercise and diet into your life and you can literally make a life changing difference.

Strength exercising will stand you in good stead as you age, it has been proven in many studies throughout the Western world that the stronger you are physically, the likelihood lessens that you will succumb to falls as you age, for it is weak muscles that usually cause us to fall, and weak bones that cause the resultant life threatening fractures.

The human body is a wonderful creation and it is very forgiving, even after many years of inactivity, it can be strengthened and improved with exercise to give a better quality of life. Medical conditions can be improved by changing dietary habits and establishing an exercise routine YOU can cope with.

In the United Kingdom it is estimated that 1 in 2 women and 1 in 5 men will suffer a bone fracture after the age of 50 at a cost to the NHS of billions each year, very often signifying the end to active life or even to life itself, depending on whether it be a hip, leg, arm or spinal fracture.

DO NOT BECOME PART OF THESE STATISTICS

MY MOTIVATION

My personal motivation was a serious illness resulting in heart valve failure in early forties and again in mid-fifties. Following successful valve replacement surgery I emerged from a long period of inactivity to find that my fitness level had deteriorated badly and middle age had set in with a vengeance. Joint stiffness, migraine headaches, a neck that would hardly move, always tired; no energy at all. I consulted a chiropractor who succeeded in temporarily relieving many of these symptoms by regular treatments and who strongly advocated walking and taking regular exercise. What me? With my headaches, aching joints, perpetual tiredness, impossible!

However, I did follow his advice to a degree and started a water aerobics class, which on reflection was really much too strenuous, and I managed to injure a hip during the class. On x-ray I was diagnosed with early osteo-arthritis, with a hip replacement forecast about 5 years hence. Back to square one. I really felt old, seeing immobility looming, thoughts of walking sticks, Zimmer frames, staggering from bed to chair, stopping on the way to take a painkiller, filled my mind. I determined then to take some action, but what? I had no idea of just what exercises I could do that could be commenced at a very modest rate and increased gradually, until I discovered strength exercise.

The wonderful thing about strength exercising is that you can start at the lowest level and provided you persevere and exercise regularly, you will improve gradually – which is the best way to go if you are in an older age group and unexercised when you commence.

I discovered through sometimes painful trial and error that unsuitable exercises, demanding too much of an unfit body can be seriously damaging and can mean months of recovery, after which you will probably never want to exercise again.

Not too much to soon must be the modus operandi.

I eventually experienced astounding success and wrote the book so that I could spread the word to YOU so that you can share in the benefits of my research and triumph over the perils of the ageing process.

My general health is much improved and many of those annoying aches and pains in joints and muscles have disappeared. Interestingly when I attended for a follow up x-ray one year after starting strength exercising, there had been no deterioration in the arthritic hip condition and I have had no further problems. Also I no longer suffer migraine headaches, but whether the latter can be attributed to exercise or is due to some other reason, I do not know and I cannot honestly claim that migraine can be cured in this way. Also, rather surprisingly, after a few weeks of exercising, my waist reappeared – which was a very welcome side issue.

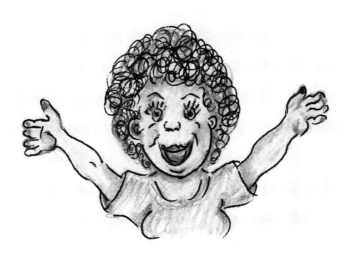

We all love a good laugh but …. did you know that laughter can diminish depression and alleviate pain and stress? A really good belly wrenching chuckle exercises nearly every organ – it's great for blood pressure too. Try it as often as possible

MAKING THE CONNECTION

MUSCLES – BONES - EXERCISE = STRENGTH

Muscle weakness was once considered to be part of growing old. We begin to lose muscle strength in early middle age, even earlier if we are sedentary. It declines by approximately 15 per cent per decade, accelerating as we reach 60's and 70's. By working the muscles, a great deal can be done to reverse this process. Exercise stimulates the blood flow and the resultant heat generated improves circulation and encourages the removal of toxic waste products from the body, allowing nutrients to be carried around the body more efficiently. One of the end results is that muscle strength and function are improved. Lack of exercise also results in cartilage shrinking. A sedentary lifestyle causes the cartilage to shrink and stiffen, reducing joint mobility. Cartilage does not have a blood supply and relies instead on synovial fluid moving in and out of the joints to nourish them and take away waste. This requires joint movement and some joint stress.

Muscles need to be taxed and then rested to grow and strengthen, If they are not worked they will be unable play their role in strengthening the body, they will weaken faster with inactivity and we will not be able to rely on strong muscles for support and to protect the bones.

Hence the importance of training the whole body, not just what we perceive to be a problem area. Muscles are linked to the bones and strength exercising will cause muscles to contract, stimulating the bones with a 'pulling' action, making the bones work too, encouraging the bone renewal process.

In a study in Scandinavia, 20 over 50 post menopausal women were invited to join a study in which they performed strength exercises for a period of six months. At the end of that period their daughters were invited to join the final class of the study; in every case, the mothers, having practised strength exercises for six months, proved stronger than their daughters. Muscles are intended to remain strong throughout life; it is inactivity, not age, which causes weakness.

Water intake is important whilst exercising, exercise depletes the muscles of water and they must be hydrated so that they can grow. Muscles actually grow following exercise, which is why there must be a day of rest between exercising each set of muscles. Keep a glass or bottle of water handy whilst exercising to keep your body topped up.

Remember
it is weak muscles
that cause falls in the elderly,
weak bones
cause the resultant fractures.

THE BONE ZONE

Low bone density or osteoporosis, has been called the silent enemy. It is very common and it usually produces no symptoms until suddenly you are prone to bone fractures, usually discovered by a fall or impact.

Osteoporosis is something of which we are all aware; it is a condition resulting from loss of bone tissue. Bone is alive and constitutes a hard outer shell with an inner 'mesh' mainly consisting of protein and minerals; living cells with their own supply of blood and nerves.   When bone density is lost the inner 'mesh' becomes more holes than bone and is consequently weakened and we become prone to fractures and breaks.

The skeleton is made up of 206 bones that are all linked together to form a strong framework, which is maintained by a healthy diet and exercise.

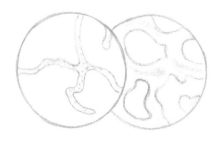

Healthy bone (left) Osteoporotic bone right.

Research shows that osteoporosis does not only attack post menopausal women, as was once thought, but men and even teenagers are also at risk. Poor diet, (bereft of essential vitamins), and lack of exercise and exposure to sun are contributory factors.

The normal ageing process causes bone loss to begin between the mid thirties and fifty years of age but an unhealthy lifestyle can mean that bone loss begins much earlier.   It has been proven that starting an exercise regime of strength exercises at any age can help reverse bone loss. Statistics have shown that resistance exercise has even benefited people in their 80's and 90's and helped them regain some independence.

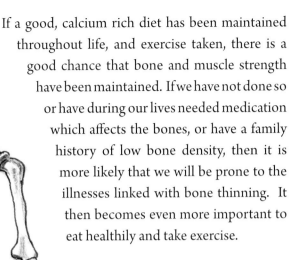

If a good, calcium rich diet has been maintained throughout life, and exercise taken, there is a good chance that bone and muscle strength have been maintained. If we have not done so or have during our lives needed medication which affects the bones, or have a family history of low bone density, then it is more likely that we will be prone to the illnesses linked with bone thinning. It then becomes even more important to eat healthily and take exercise.

By the age of 65 men have lost approximately 10 per cent of their bone mass and women at the same age 26 per cent. Strength exercising involving the whole body is the best way to combat this, combined with a healthy diet. As bone and muscles are linked, using weights to strengthen muscles also works the bones and strengthens them too. Bone is living tissue and changes constantly throughout life, as old bone is broken down (osteoclast activity) and renewal takes place (osteoblast activity.) However, as we age, the osteoblast activity slows, increasingly with each decade. Undertaking strength exercise and a calcium rich diet encourages bone to replenish again.

There are other important uses for calcium and if the diet is lacking in this mineral, it will be drawn from the bones to fulfil other needs, so bones become even more frail.

By providing the correct nutrients and exercise, bone renewal is encouraged and the bone mass can grow – a process that must be maintained if we are to remain strong.

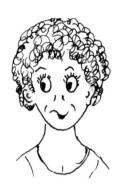

Calcium is a multi-tasking mineral and also assists in the following:-
Blood Clotting
Controlling Cholesterol Levels
Controlling Muscle and Nerve
Contractions via the Brain
Maintaining Heart Function
Sleep Patterns

Osteoporosis can very often be prevented and once diagnosed can be helped by medication, improved calcium intake and strength exercise.

We are never quite sure how much of the calcium taken naturally in our diet actually arrives at the bones, but it has been suggested from studies that calcium absorption can be more efficient when it is obtained from plants, not from dairy products, but the quantities needed are high and are probably difficult to achieve for most people.   Exercise will assist in calcium absorption, not intensive aerobic exercise, but particularly strength exercise, carried out regularly. Vitamin D obtained from sunshine is very important, in the bone building process and we should, whenever possible spend 20 minutes or so each day in the sun, if this is not possible, and in our climate much of the year is bereft of sun, then a vitamin D supplement could be considered.

Using a sunscreen higher than Factor 6 can inhibit absorption of sunlight. Essential calcium is abundant in dairy products.

Some of the best calcium sources are listed below. The over 50's need between 1000 and 1200 mg. per day. A typical day's requirement could include any of the following to attain 1200 mg.:-

1 cup of low fat fortified milk	300 mg.
1 low fat yogurt	300 mg.
Sardines, with bones, no salt	325 mg.
Pilchards with bones	300 mg.
1 Cup of Spinach	295 mg.
3 oz. Tofu with added calcium	100 mg.
1 oz. of Almonds	71 mg.
1 cup of Soya milk with added calcium	300 mg.
3 oz. Rainbow trout	144 mg.
3 oz. Tinned salmon with bones	120 mg.
Tofu	90 mg.
Curly Kale (cooked)	85 mg.
1 cup of Calcium fortified orange juice	350 mg.
Cheddar Cheese 1.4 oz.	307 mg.
Blue Cheese 1.5 oz.	225 mg.

If you do choose to obtain your calcium from sources other than dairy products, make sure that you are eating masses of green vegetables, almonds, seeds and pulses and foods offering a source of calcium, also oily fish, such as sardines (with bones) and salmon. If you wish to drink milk but avoid dairy products, substitute Soya products containing added calcium and vitamins. So Good is our favourite milk substitute, produced from Soya protein; it is great for building strong bones and helps to lower cholesterol and maintain a healthy heart. It is delicious on breakfast cereals and can be used for making sauces, custards and as a drink or smoothie (yummy with honey for a sleep inducing late night drink.)

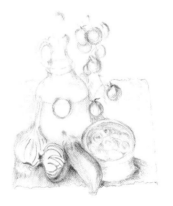

Garlic, olive oil and onions form a large part of the Mediterranean diet and are thought to be part of the reason why the area has a lower incidence of heart disease and cancer than elsewhere in the west.

WHAT ARE STRENGTH EXERCISES

and
WHAT IS THE DIFFERENCE BETWEEN STRENGTH EXERCISE AND WEIGHT BEARING & RESISTANCE EXERCISE?

WEIGHT BEARING EXERCISES

Are those in which your bones and muscles work against gravity.   It can be any exercises in which your feet and legs are bearing your weight e.g. walking, dancing, tennis, stair climbing.

RESISTANCE EXERCISE

Means working against an opposing force (i.e. a weight).

STRENGTH EXERCISES

Are a combination of both the above and you are more likely these days to find weight bearing and resistance exercises referred to as Strength Exercises.

We favour the use of free weights (hand weights) because they involve the whole body to facilitate balance and concentration/control. For example, working the back, shoulders and chest also works the arms, wrists and hands, legs and feet. All parts of the body come into play as you control posture, breathing and balance. Always commence your exercises as they are set out, it is important that the back muscles are strengthened first, followed by chest, shoulders, arms. Strong back muscles are essential for they have a great deal of work to do. Do not overwork any one set of muscles, it is counter productive and you will regret it next day when you experience aches and pains. Work only until the last two repeats of a particular exercise become difficult. Strength is gained gradually by working each set of muscles in turn.

STRENGTH EXERCISE is also a very effective way to reduce your body fat, for as fat reduces, lean muscle mass will increase and muscle has a higher energy need than fat tissue, so as you replace fat tissue with muscle, the calories will burn. You will of course also be building up bone density.

STRENGTH EXERCISE, undertaken on a regular basis will tone up and build muscle and increase bone density. You need to exercise each set of muscles three times each week, whether you split the programme and work one day on the back, chest and shoulders, and the next day the abdominals, arms, hips, legs and ankles is up to you, but give each set of muscles a day of rest, as they grow and strengthen on the rest day, not actually during exercise.

However, regularity is of prime importance, if you only exercise once each week you will be starting anew each time and will not make progress.

Do not worry that you will gain bulk by using weights, you will not be progressing beyond say, 5 Kg., it will tone & build muscles also strengthening your bones. Strength exercising is a very efficient way to look slimmer, toned and more sculpted, besides improving balance.

WARM UP BEFORE YOU START

Always commence your strength exercise session with a warm up, this means that your blood will be warm when you start, and make strength exercising easier. If you work cold muscles they can suffer tiny tears in tissue and boy, will you know about it next day!

Warming up can be walking on a treadmill, sweeping the terrace, vacuuming the house, cleaning the car, dancing around the house to your favourite music, swimming, it all counts as warming up and walking the dog for 30 minutes uses the same amount of energy as playing tennis for 12 minutes.

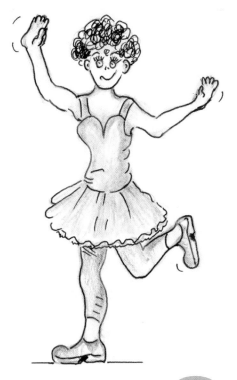

DIET AWARENESS

Exercise and diet are two things over which we have total control, we can decide to opt for a healthy diet, take an interest in the goodness derived to help the body to age well by eating foods rich in vitamins and minerals;   or totally ignore the quality of the food we eat, disregarding the fact that it may be actually doing harm.

SALT

We are warned that a high salt intake can cause high blood pressure, heart problems, strokes; it will also leach calcium from the bones, increasing bone frailty. The recommended consumption is up to 6g per day. In this country, we are thought to each consume around 12g. A pinch of salt is about 0.25g whilst a teaspoon is 5g.   A bag of crisps can contain as much as 2.8g. A slice of bread will contain about ½g salt, therefore 6 slices of bread will give you half of your daily salt consumption in one go! Instant cup-a-soup contains up to 2.5g salt and tinned and carton varieties are heavy in salt too. A medium sized pizza will give the whole days RDA in one meal!   Many breakfast cereals contain more salt than a packet of crisps, Shredded Wheat is an exception, containing only a trace of salt. Convenience foods are very high in salt.

The following lists some everyday foods which are high in salt, so try to avoid them, replacing with healthier foods.

Bacon. Ham. Tongue. Sausage. Salami. Salt Beef. Sausage. Meat pates. Burgers. Tinned vegetables. Tinned and packet soups. Cheese. Butter (use unsalted.) Crisps. Biscuits. Salted nuts. Some breakfast cereals. Smoked fish. Malted drinks. Most pies and pasties. Meat extracts. Most bottled sauces. Most ready meals.

Some supermarkets now offer clearer labelling showing the recommended daily salt intake and the salt content of a particular food or drink.

If you are used to a high salt intake you may find at first that food tastes bland without it, but your palate will adjust in about two weeks and you will then begin to taste the food! Season your food with herbs or try a seasoning salt that contains sea salt, and various dried herbs, excellent for soups and casseroles.

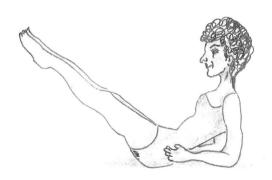

Do not eat last thing at night. Your digestive system really feels the strain of this extra burden – it needs to rest too and recuperate from a hard day's work.
AND… … ..
remember that the liver detoxes whilst it is NOT working in the early hours. It is a good idea to aid it (and extend it's life) by being in bed asleep by midnight.

SEASONING WITHOUT SALT

When roasting, pan cooking or grilling, use olive oil and mix in with a couple of tablespoons of balsamic vinegar, a wonderful aroma and delicious taste.

Add a little mint to potatoes and vegetables when cooking.

Spread mustard lightly on beef about two thirds of the time through roasting.

Add wholegrain mustard to mashed potatoes.

Sprinkle a little cinnamon on pork during cooking or add to apple sauce.

When roasting lamb, cut several deep slits in the meat and tuck a sprig of rosemary and a clove of garlic in each one.

Cut slits into potatoes prior to roasting and push in snippets of garlic.

Place sprigs of tarragon around chicken and then cook.

Add chives to mashed potatoes and also to omelettes, soups and salads.

Use bay leaves in marinades, stock and rice dishes (remove prior to serving.)

Tomatoes, egg dishes, mushrooms and French dressing are improved with a sprinkling of basil.

Sprinkle lemon juice on vegetables prior to serving.

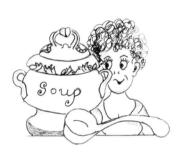

Hattie's Hints
Give your digestive system a rest from time to time and spend a whole day just drinking home made soups, fruit and vegetable juices and glasses of water.

Tomatoes are full of antioxidants and are even healthier when cooked, tinned tomatoes are equally good.
Research now shows that the rich lycopene source of tomatoes helps the bone replacement cycle as well as helping in the prevention of cancer.

WATER - HOW MUCH SHOULD WE DRINK?

We lose around 6 pints daily in natural bodily functions and we should put in excess of that amount back to have full energy. Aim for 2.5 litres, fill a drinking bottle and keep it with you at all times throughout the day. It reminds you to drink and it's there close to hand!

The body is 75% water and a loss of only 3% can cause a loss of physical energy and mental strength. This is often mistaken for hunger and a quick fix snack is ought. Unfortunately this does not fix anything and 15 minutes later you will be feeling just as drear. Drink 2 or 3 glasses of water instead to re-hydrate your body and you will feel instantly more alert and less tired. Starting the day with a large glass of water will cleanse your system; a glass of water mid morning and mid afternoon will avoid the lowering of your energy level. A large glass of water taken at night will help cleanse your system and help you settle down for sleep.

Water is a multi-tasking agent and it cannot work efficiently if there is not enough available when the body makes its demands. It is necessary for the following functions:-

Lubrication of joints
Carrying nutrients around the body
Pancreatic function
Transporting waste products of cells through the body
Lubrication of the colon ~ Saliva ~ Muscle hydration
Working with nutrients to volumise
the muscles following exercise ~ Skin hydration

It is not surprising that we can feel so low and out of sorts if we neglect our water intake. Early signs of dehydration are often signalled by the following symptoms:-

Dry skin
Headaches
Constipation
Tiredness
Strong urine i.e. a darker colour than straw

When exercising always carry a bottle of water with you.

Although several drinks may be taken during the day, if they are loaded with caffeine, alcohol or additives, they will aid dehydration. The skin ages more quickly if you do not drink sufficient water. When hydrated it will plump up, lines and wrinkles become less prominent and dark circles under the eyes decrease.

That tired, low feeling that hits around early afternoon is often a sign of dehydration, not hunger. Instead of a 'quick fix' chocolate bar, try a large glass of water for a real lift.

Bone density is not aided by drinking fizzy water; it contains high levels of phosphate (phosphoric acid) which strips the bones of calcium.

Equal levels of calcium and phosphorous are naturally maintained in our bodies, so if we drink an excess of carbonated drinks, the precious calcium is leached from the bones to correct the balance.

If you do not wish to drink tap water, buy still, bottled water. Many people feel that bottled water is safer, but this is not necessarily so. Purchasing masses of bottles at a time is not a good idea. Store bottled water in the fridge and treat as you would any fresh food.

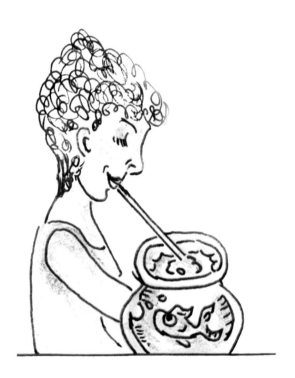

HATTIE'S HINT
For every drink of alcohol or caffeine taken in a day, drink an extra glass of water.
If you have a hangover, several glasses of water and a brisk walk in the fresh air will work wonders.

LIFE'S ESSENTIALS

VITAMINS AND MINERALS

These are the things that will keep the body functioning; digesting and eliminating food, circulating oxygen, assisting in the function of all organs, keeping bones and muscles strong, giving mental alertness, clear skin, bright eyes, general good health and a zest for life. Ideally they will be obtained from the food we eat if we make sure that it is good food, not just a token meal, merely assuaging hunger.

Vitamins and minerals are one of the most important tools we have to fight the ageing process, another being exercise. The foods that you introduce to your body will either assist it to fight off disease and ageing, determining HOW you age, or they will do the opposite and aid the ageing process.

Vitamins and minerals protect the body from disease and ageing. Ideally a wide variety of both should be included in the daily diet. They will all work together and ensure that the blood, organs, digestion, and elimination process, brain cells, bones and muscles are fed nutritionally and can perform their functions well. By enriching the diet in this way we cannot help but be healthier, and this also reflects in appearance with clearer skin and brighter eyes, strong nails and shiny hair. It is thought that a high proportion of adult cancers may be preventable, many being due to the deficiencies of the western diet, which can be rectified by eating more fresh foods such as fruit and vegetables. In addition a high vitamin intake will make you less likely to succumb to infections, such as common colds and flu.

If food intake consists of prepared and fast foods, the body, to process the preservatives, chemicals and saturated fats, contained will be working overtime. In fact it hardly stops. A high fat meal for instance, can stay in the digestive system for almost 20 hours, during that time it is fermenting and producing toxins that have to be dealt with. We will of course feel tired after a heavy meal and is it any wonder that such a diet will accelerate ageing? The stomach, pancreas, liver and kidneys are all working so hard that their life is shortening and they are not getting nutrition from the food to assist their functions. The results are what we have now become to accept as normal when we age, high blood pressure, high cholesterol, arthritis and lethargy. However, fresh food, fruit and vegetables are assimilated and processed quickly by the body and the internal organs can then take a rest until the next meal comes along.

It is wise to limit your intake of saturated fats (mainly found in animal products and processed foods) and avoid anything labelled hydrogenated fats (these are the ones that are solid at room temperature, e.g. margarines) and are contained in many ready made foods, cakes and pastries, potato crisps, chocolate bars. These fats have been chemically treated to increase shelf life and can be harmful, apart from having no nutritional value at all. Use olive oil for roasting and frying, it is a natural product and does not undergo harmful changes when heated.

We need an abundance of vitamins and minerals in the diet to keep healthy and look good. If we seriously want to improve health and appearance, it is very easy to make a choice. Study a pack of convenience food and note the ingredients. Is it rich in vitamins and minerals? Will it provide anti-oxidants? How much fat and preservative does it contain? How much salt and sugar? What will you gain from eating it, apart from weight?

Now take just one medium apple. It is a powerful source of nutrients, including potassium, folic acid, Vitamin C and calcium, traces of B vitamins, carotene, iron, magnesium and zinc. There is no saturated fat or cholesterol and it has around 80 calories to sustain you. Consider one carrot, it contains Vitamins C, D and niacin, pyridoxine, folic acid, biotin, Pantothenic acid, potassium, sodium, copper, calcium and magnesium.

Moving on to green, leafy vegetables, kale for instance will provide Vitamins A & C, manganese, copper, tryptophan, calcium, Vitamin B6, potassium, foliate, phosphorus, Vitamin B3 (in order of density).

Is there a difficult choice to make? We don't think so, not if healthy eating is the aim. The apple, carrot and kale win hands down.

SOME ESSENTIAL ~VITAMINS AND MINERALS, SOME OF THEIR FUNCTIONS & SOURCES

A (Retinol).　Sources: - Oatmeal, Dairy Products, Egg yolk, Mackerel, Spinach, Whole grains, Mango, Oranges, Melon, Cabbage, Potatoes, Broccoli, Beef, Liver.

Assists: - Skin, bone and tooth growth, vision, immunity and reproduction.

B1 (Thiamine) Sources:- Oatmeal, Pork, Milk, vegetables, seafood, sunflower seeds, brown rice.

Aids metabolism and nerve functions.

B2 (Riboflavin) Sources: - Milk, eggs, green vegetables, fish, whole grains

Aids energy, metabolism, normal vision and skin health

B3 (Niacin)　Sources: - Salmon, tuna, eggs, milk, avocados, sunflower seeds, lean meats.

Gives energy, helps maintain metabolism, skin health, nervous system and digestive system

B12 (Cyancobalamin)

> Sources: - Milk, meat, eggs, fish.

> Used in new cell manufacture, nerve cell maintenance helps break down fatty and amino acids,

B5 (Pantothenic acid)

> Sources: - Beef, liver whole grains, nuts. eggs, Green vegetables.

> Anti-stress Converts carbohydrates to energy

B6 (Pyridoxin)

> Sources: - Pork, Beef, Fortified Cereals, Oatmeal, Bananas. Eggs, Milk, Avocados, Seeds, Soya Products.

> Assists:- Amino acid and fatty acid metabolism, red blood cell production

C

> Sources: - Citrus Fruits, Kiwi. Blueberries, Sweet Potatoes, Broccoli, Brussels sprouts, Legumes, Green Pepper, Leafy Vegetables,

> An antioxidant helps immunity, iron absorption

D

> Sources: - Milk, Egg yolk, Sardines, Salmon, Mackerel, Tuna, Beans Sunshine.

> Assists bone maintenance

E.

> Sources: - Leafy Green Vegetables, Wheat germ, Broccoli, Eggs, Oats, Butter, Peanuts, Seeds, Vegetable Oils, Milk, Olive Oil, Soya Products.

> An Antioxidant supports cell maintenance

K

Sources: - Live yogurt. Broccoli, Spinach,
Leafy Green vegetables, Cheese, Green Tea.

Aids- manufacture of blood clotting proteins.
Cell maintenance

Biotin

Sources:- Lamb, Dairy Products, Egg Yolks, Nuts.

Assists:- Nerves, Skin growth & health . Energy

Boron

Sources: - Tomatoes, Apples, Pears, Raisins, Pulses.

Aids: - Bone and muscle health

Calcium

Sources: - Dairy Products, Soya Products, Salmon, Sardines,
Root Vegetables, Green Leafy Vegetables, Broccoli,
Broad Beans, Sesame Seeds.

Aids: - Bone growth & maintenance. Blood Clotting.
Brain Function Control of Cholesterol Levels.
Control of Muscle and Nerve Contractions Maintaining
Heart Function Sleep Patterns

Carotene

Sources: - Dark leafy greens, Broccoli, Orange coloured fruit
and vegetables (carrots, apricots).

Aids: - Antioxidant. Thought to prevent cancer
and useful in Rheumatoid arthritis

Chromium

Sources: - Milk, Fruit Egg Yolk, Mushrooms,
Root Vegetables, Green Leafy Vegetables

Stimulates insulin activity.

Choline   Sources: - Egg Yolk, Beef, Soya products

                 Helps nerve impulses, Helps maintain cell structure.
                 Helps nerve energy (memory function)
                 helps metabolise fats and cholesterol.

Copper   Sources: - Avocado, Shellfish, Whole Grains, Fruits

                 Aids: - Adrenal hormones. Helps iron absorption
                 Maintains blood and connective tissues

Cobalt   Sources:- Meat, Fruit Leafy Vegetables, Milk.

                 Assists: - B12 in production of red blood cells.
                 Helps maintain the nervous system

Fluoride   Sources: - Seafood, Meat, Black Tea, Added to most tap water.

                 Supplements should not be taken
                 without consulting a physician

Folic Acid   Sources:-:- Eggs, Wheat germ, Leafy Green Vegetables

                 Aids: - Red blood cell formation. Division of blood cells
                 Division of body cells.

Insitol   Sources: - Citrus fruits, Wheat germ, Melon, Peanuts.

                 Aids: - Brain cell function. Helps liver function

Iodine   Seafood, meat, Black tea.

                 Produces hormones from the thyroid gland.
                 May help prevent heart disease

Iron	Shellfish, Nuts, broccoli, red meat Egg Yolk.
	Assists: - Production of haemoglobin. Immune activity. liver function.
Magnesium	Sources: - Pulses (e.g. Soya beans) Brown rice, whole grain
	Supports bone mineralisation, protein building, muscular contraction, nerve impulse transmission, immunity
Manganese	Sources: - Leafy Vegetables, Root Vegetables, Nuts, Cereals.
	Helps brain function and antioxidant. Metabolises calcium.
Molybdenum	Sources:- Wheat germ, eggs, liver.
	Utilises iron. Thought to help prevent cancer.
Omega 3&6 Fatty Acids	Sources: - Oily fish, (salmon, mackerel, sardines) flax, walnuts, pumpkin seeds, whole grain bread, whole grain seeds, breakfast cereals, (Shredded Wheat, Weetabix), sunflower seeds, hemp seeds, Organic free range eggs.
	Assists:- Production of cell membranes, regulates blood pressure, heart rate, protects vital organs, essential to body function.
Potassium	Sources: - Avocados, Leafy Green Vegetables, Bananas, Potatoes, Nuts
	Maintains fluid and electrolyte balance, cell integrity, muscle contractions and nerve impulse transmission. Helps normalise blood pressure.

Phosphorous   Sources:- Meat, Fish, Cheese, Soya Products.

                  Helps form bones, teeth & cell membranes.
                  Boosts endurance

Selenium   Sources: - Tuna, Onions, Whole-wheat Bread,
                  Tomatoes, Wheat germ, Broccoli.

                  Antioxidant Skin, hair, eyesight boosts liver function.
                  Boosts immune system Protects against circulatory
                  diseases and thought to be anti-ageing. Aids detoxification.

Vanadium   Sources: - Parsley, Lettuce, Radish, Olive Oil,
                  Dairy Products, Fruit.

                  Thought to be anti cholesterol & high blood pressure

Zinc   Sources: - Meat, Mushrooms, Seeds & Nuts, Eggs,
                  Wholegrain Bread, Wheat germ.

                  Antioxidant. Immunity. Growth, energy metabolism ,
                  Haemoglobin

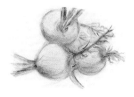

HATTIE'S HINTS
Recently published information regarding Blood Pressure
claims that drinking 500 ml. of Beetroot Juice every day
will reduce blood pressure. Within 2 hours blood pressure reduces
for at least 24 hours.

WHAT IS A PORTION?

Recommended portion sizes are:-

Vegetables = 3 heaped tablespoons

salad – 1 dessert bowl

medium sized fruit
e.g. apple, pear, kiwi, banana = 1 fruit

very large fruit
e.g. melon, pineapple = 1 large slice

large fruit
e.g. grapefruit, mango, papayas = 1 fruit

small fruits,
e.g. plums, apricots, Satsuma's = 2 fruits

small fruits
e.g. raspberries, strawberries, blueberries, grapes = 1 mug

vegetable juice (home made) = 1 glass (150 ml.)
One cup (approx 100g) of raw greens
½ cup beans or peas

HATTIE'S HINTS

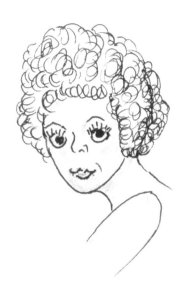

Organic Cider Vinegar is reputed to be useful in alleviating rheumatoid arthritis by helping break down uric acid crystals in the joints, to be taken three times a day with honey in hot water. Accompany with Epsom salts baths or a sauna, twice each day, to assist in eliminating these nasties from the body.

Many fruit and vegetables can be juiced, which also provides the benefit of using the raw, uncooked product so that virtually no nutrients are lost in preparation. Carrot and/or apple juice are an excellent combination and a good basis for many vegetable juices, broccoli or kale can be added, and herbs can be included to give an extra zing to the taste.

A few suggestions for juicing are:-
A cupful of broccoli or kale with 2 kiwi fruit and an apple.
3 large tomatoes, a handful of parsley and a few sprigs of basil will give a juice with an Italian zing.
A sliver of ginger added to two carrots, a handful of broccoli or kale, a large tomato, makes an excellent juice.
2 Sticks of celery, a handful of spinach, 3 apples and a pear.
A handful of strawberries or raspberries, 2 pears.
Try juicing a pineapple, delicious, smooth and creamy.

Experiment with a wide variety of fruits and vegetables and do not be afraid to mix the two. We have tried dozens of combinations and not found anything we dislike.

When you purchase a juicer, look for one with a large enough feeder to take large portions such as whole fruits & vegetables e.g. apples and pears, carrots. Just wash, no need to peel and chop. A stem of broccoli can be cut into three pieces and easily juiced. So much more convenient than chopping everything into tiny portions and you will be much more inclined to use it. Do not keep your juicer tucked away in a cupboard, let it live on the worktop in full view, you are not likely to forget its existence or feel you cannot be bothered to find it, put it together and then use it.

Drink juiced fruit and vegetables immediately as vitamins are depleted within 20 minutes.

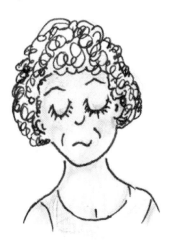

For a sleep inducing late night drink take a glass of warmed milk (use a Soya substitute if you are intolerant to cow's milk) and add a tablespoon of honey

MAKING THE COMMITMENT

PRIOR TO PLANNING YOUR START INTO A NEW LIFE OF EXERCISE, BEWARE OF OBSTACLES YOU MAY NEED TO OVERCOME

Committing to an exercise regime is often the most difficult part. We have all, throughout our lives, started with the best of intentions and then after a week or so, something more important or far more interesting has 'popped up' and we have missed our class or session in the gym or it is not a convenient time at home to set aside an hour or so to exercise. Suddenly the reasons for doing it in the first place become obscure and we decide that after all it's not for us, we don't need it really, do we? So we give up.

Be warned that your mind can go into overdrive establishing excellent excuses why you should not work out today, BUT tomorrow can quickly become NEVER. We are incredibly clever at doing this and can easily convince ourselves that exercise is a waste of time and go comfortably on in our inactive lifestyle. One good way to avoid this is to always arrange a firm time and place to exercise with a friend, you will not want to let your friend down and it will work equally well for her/him. It is a great incentive. Be determined to improve your everyday life and health for the rest of your life.

Possible obstacles to be overcome:-

I DON'T HAVE TIME

There are 24 hours in each day. Prioritise your day and put health first on your agenda.

I'M TOO OLD

Even at 90 you can improve your fitness level with moderate weight bearing and resistance exercise.

I'M TOO TIRED
Exercise will give you extra energy

I HATE THE GYM
You can actually do it all at home.

I AM ARTHRITIC, EXERCISE HURTS MY JOINTS.
They will improve with regular exercise

I HAVE TOO MANY ACHES AND PAINS TO EVEN THINK ABOUT IT.

It can only get better and will be worth the effort.

To exercise painful joints and muscles is something we usually feel we do not want to do, but becoming active gradually over a period of time is the only way to achieve an improvement. Our personal experience of this amazed us, we could not believe the increase in mobility and flexibility of joints and the strength gained in muscles.

Prior to starting, it seems much more enticing to dine out, enjoying a good lunch or dinner, a few glasses of your favourite vino and then home to read a book or watch TV., feet up, relaxing , perhaps zzzzzzzzzing a few hours away. When you begin to feel the energising effect of exercising and the benefits start to kick in, you will want to do this only when you have exercised – you will be anxious to maintain your progress.

If you are exercising at home, it is possible to improvise using a chair, stools, a staircase, but some of the exercises are easier performed on an exercise bench and you can purchase one from Argos, for instance for around £40.00 and also sets of weights can be purchased in the High Street for between £12 and £20.00.

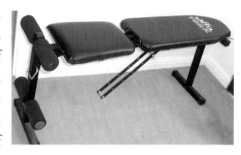

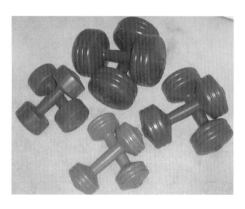

These sets of weights will begin at ½ Kg and go up to 5 Kg, which should be sufficient for your purpose.

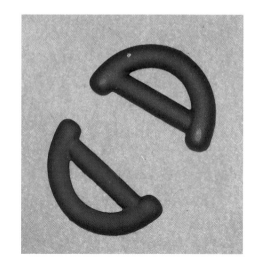

We find this 'D' type of weight very easy to use and when we last checked, Tesco (the Hypermarket store) were selling them individually from ½ Kg upwards.

SETS AND REPEATS EXPLAINED

A set is defined as the same exercise repeated several times. e.g. Abdominals. The Abdominal Crunch repeated 10 times equals one set. A further 10 repeats completes another set.

It is important to establish the correct technique and use weights of a size that is comfortable. Start modestly, you can only improve. The number of repeats should be governed by your fitness. When the repeats become harder, (work ONLY UNTIL the last two repeats are difficult) you will know that you have reached your current limit. When all the repeats become easy, it is time to increase the weight OR increase the repeats, – Not both at the same time.

DO NOT WORK ON TO FAILURE OR EXHAUSTION

Aim to complete one set of 10 repeats as your starting point. If you are totally unexercised, start with the lightest weight and do only 5 repeats until you feel it is getting easier. You are not in competition; you have only your own fitness to consider and there is no deadline.

TAKE IT SLOWLY

Work carefully, control your breathing and perfect your technique.

When you increase the weights, you may need to reduce the number of repeats and build up again slowly. You may find that some days you can do more than others, which is fine. If you do feel really energised, carry on and do another set of repeats. Make a note of your progress, chart your repeats, and you will be surprised at the improvement made.

Wear comfortable, loose clothing, nothing to restrict your movements and something supportive and comfortable on your feet.

TAKE NOTE

If you are elderly, totally unexercised (at any age) or if you have existing health problems, are taking medication or are doubtful of your suitability for the exercises, consult your medical practitioner prior to commencing this, or any exercise programme, or making dietary changes, or taking supplements.

If you are elderly, have health problems or are totally unexercised, make sure that you are not alone when you exercise, you may need a little help from time to time.

Any exercise or dietary advice given in this book is not intended to replace any advice or medication given by your medical advisor.

If you feel dizzy or unwell or are in pain during the exercise, stop and take a rest, if it happens again, stop and seek medical advice prior to recommencing.

If you are new to exercising or want to make it as easy as possible, split the exercise session into two parts and exercise different muscles on consecutive days. DO NOT exercise the same muscles on consecutive days, they need a day of rest to grow and strengthen. For example you could work the upper and lower back, the abdomen and chest on day one and on day two, work the shoulders arms, hips, legs, ankles and feet.

If you decide to carry out the exercises in one session, add an extra 5 minutes cardio vascular exercise in the middle of the programme.

Always warm up prior to exercising and always cool down afterwards. e.g. if you are walking for a warm up, slow down for the last 3 minutes and stroll. These exercises, performed regularly, three times each week is ideal, will gradually enable you to strengthen your whole body, please do them in the order shown in the examples, it is important that you commence with back strengthening, you will find that a strong back will help you to easily accomplish exercises for the smaller muscle groups. It does help if you can persuade a friend to join you. You can then compare notes and also check on each other's progress and accuracy; exercising is rather like driving, we start off well but can become sloppy in technique, almost without realising it.

These exercises do not need to be carried out in a gym; they can easily be done at home, using hand weights. Any of the exercises shown using gym equipment have alternatives that can be done at home.

To exercise painful joints and muscles is something we usually feel we do not want to do, but becoming active gradually over a period of time is the only way to achieve an improvement. My personal experience of this amazed me, I could not believe the increase in mobility and flexibility of joints and the strength gained in muscles.

A gym setting has been used for photography for ease of production. You do not necessarily need to use a bench or even weights, you could improvise with a chair, bed, or step and use cans from the larder, held in plastic bags for weights. However, you will find it easier to use the correct equipment, and the easier it is, the more likely you are to continue!

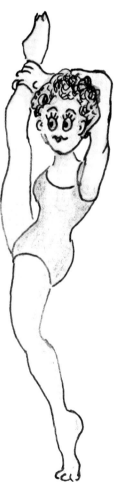

Remember:-
NEVER ATTEMPT
TOO MUCH TOO SOON

THE EXERCISES

A good stretch prior to starting will loosen up the muscles.

Tower of Pisa
Stretch Start

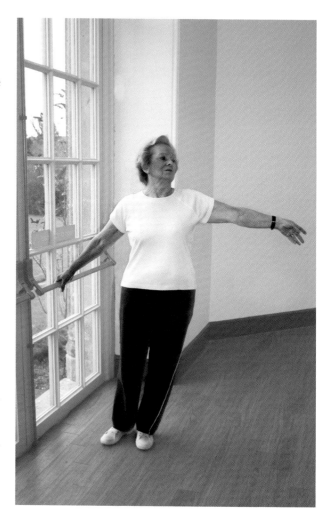

1. Stand with the right hand holding a bar (a door frame or handle will do the job too).

2. Lean away from the frame, stretching the whole body from the feet upwards.

3. Turn the body slightly to the left and stretch the left arm out away from the body.

5. Hold for a count of 3.

Repeat three times and then changeover to the left side.

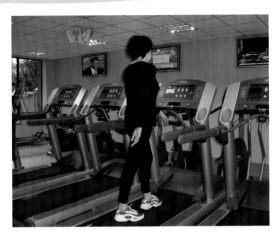

1 Start walking slowly and establish your rhythm. Walk at your own pace, you are not in a competition and your walking speed should not be influenced by the person on the neighboring treadmill. Increase and vary the speed and gradient if you want to or, simply walk at one speed for your chosen time, increasing speed over a period. You should be walking hard enough to become a little puffed, but still be able to talk. For the final 5 minutes, slow gradually to cool down. Finally, take a rest for a few minutes and drink a glass of water.

You may find slight aches and pains in feet, ankles and knees as you

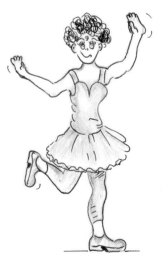

are walking but you should be able to walk through these and they should soon disappear. If the pain persists or is intense, stop. Do not be tempted to run or jog, there is no need.

The same applies to any cardio vascular exercise you choose, be it walking the dog, vacuuming the house or sweeping the yard, and if none of these appeal, dance around the house to your favourite music.

You should know when your cardio vascular rate is rising by an increasing warmth throughout your body.

WORKING THE LOWER BACK
THE PELVIC TILT

1   *Lie on your back with knees bent and feet flat on the floor.*

2   *Tighten your abdominal muscles towards your back and clench your pelvic muscles (these are the ones you would use if you are dying to spend a penny and cannot find a loo).*

3   *BREATHE IN.*

4   *BREATHING OUT, raise your pelvis slightly off the ground and hold for 5 seconds.*

5   *BREATHING IN, lower to starting position.*

6   *Repeat 10 times. This completes one set.*

7   *Repeat Set.*

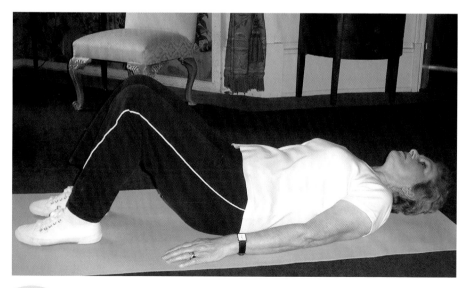

EXERCISE 3 — WORKING THE LOWER BACK
THE BRIDGE

1   Lie on your back, legs bent at the knees, feet planted hip width apart.

2   BREATHE IN.

3   BREATHING OUT, raise hips by pushing down evenly on both legs to form a bridge with the lower body .

4   Hold for a count of three and slowly lower.

5   Repeat 10 - 15 times. This completes one set.

6   Repeat Set.

7   You can extend this lift gradually until you actually lift off the ground up to shoulder level.

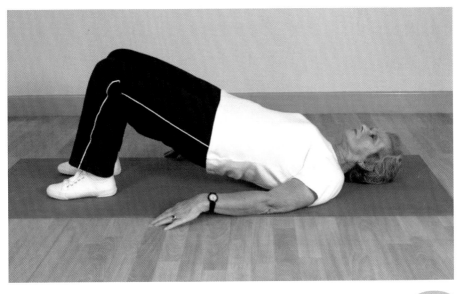

EXERCISE 4 — *WORKING THE LOWER BACK*
LOWER BACK STRETCHER

1 *Lie on your front with forehead on the floor.*

2 *Arms straight out in front of you and legs straight out behind you and BREATHE IN.*

3 *BREATHING OUT, raise your left leg and right arm 2-3 inches from the floor, simultaneously, stretching away from your body, as though stretching for something just out of reach.*

4 *Slowly relax down again.*

5 *Switch to left arm and right leg and repeat.*

Repeat 15 times on each side. Add a further set when possible.

Do not lift higher than 2-3 inches;

your efforts must be concentrated in stretching out away from your body, not upwards.

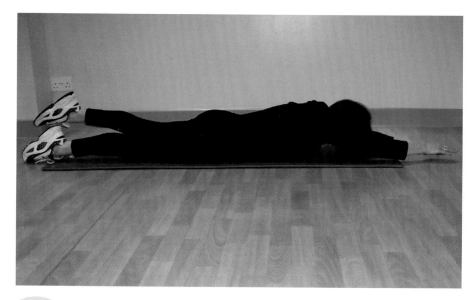

Hidden Benefits

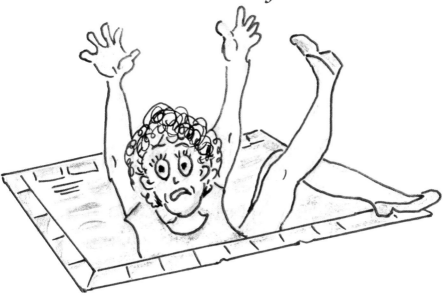

About twelve months after starting training, Pat had the misfortune to fall into a manhole in her garden which had been left uncovered by workmen.

Scratched, cut and bruised, she literally was up to her neck in trouble. There was no one home to come to her rescue and she faced the prospect of a cold night in the hole. However, remembering all her strength training, she attempted to lever herself upwards, using the newly gained strength in her shoulders and arms and was eventually successful and popped out and was able to call the emergency services to tend her injuries.

She was very aware that without strength training there was no way she would have escaped.

Proceed carefully if you have lower back problems and always do the lower back exercises first.

If performing this exercise at home, the edge of the bath, covered by a towel to prevent slipping is a good place to use.

1   *Kneel with right knee on the bench.*

2   *Hold a weight in your left hand.*

3   *Bend forward from the hips, keeping the back in a straight line, left arm straight at your side holding the weight.*

4   *Rest right hand at the furthest end of the bench for support.*

5   *BREATHE IN.*

6   *BREATHING OUT, bend the elbow slowly, lifting the weight towards your waist as far as you can.*

7   *Slowly return to the starting position.*

8   *Repeat 10 times.*

9   *Change hands, change legs. Repeat.*

10   *This completes one set*
     Repeat the set.

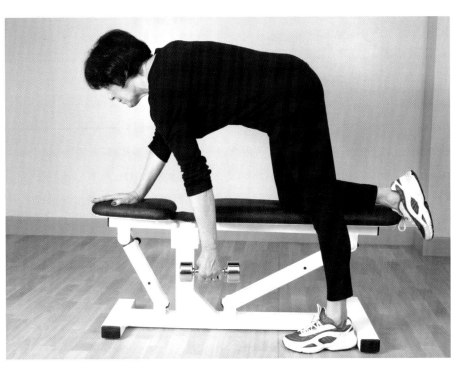

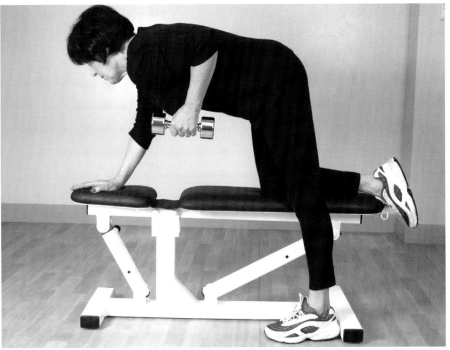

WORKING THE UPPER BACK
THE LATERAL PULL DOWN

An alternative to the Upper Back Lift. Take advantage of this equipment if you are using a gym, it's great for strengthening the upper back and will also work your shoulders and inner arms.

Adjust to your required weight (you will probably want to start with nothing more than 10 Kg). Note the bar should be pulled down in front of your body, do not attempt to pull it down behind your neck.

1   *Sit on the seat provided and adjust the knee pads to sit snugly on the tops of knees.*

2   *Reaching up, grasp the bar firmly, using the overhand grip, with hands about 3 inches in from the ends. Keep the chest lifted and lean back slightly from the hips. BREATHE IN.*

3   *BREATHING OUT, pull the bar down slowly and smoothly until level with the collar bone.*

4   *Slowly and smoothly, raise the bar back to the starting position.*

5   *Repeat 10 times. This completes one set.*

6   *Repeat set.*

Do not bend the wrists.
Do not pull down the bar beyond the collar bone.
Do not lean back.
Do not move the head backwards as you pull down.

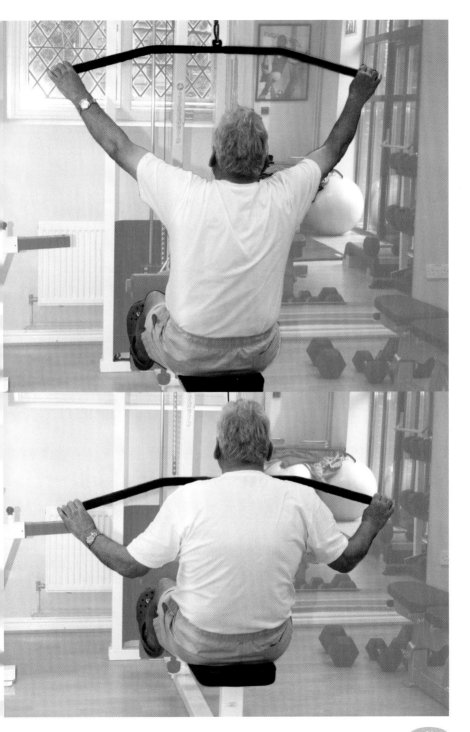

WORKING THE UPPER BACK
THE PULLOVER

This exercise will give your back, arms, shoulders, neck, chest and abdomen a fantastic stretch and is wonderful if you have neck or shoulder tension. Make sure that your head is supported. Be careful if you have lower back problems.

The exercise can be performed on the floor, taking the weight behind your head to rest on the floor. If you are unexercised, elderly or unsure of your ability, perform the exercise in this way first, until your lower back strengthens.

1   *Lie on the bench with feet supported on the floor*
      or on the bar of the bench.

2   *Tighten the abdominals*
      (this will help strengthen the lower back muscles).

3   *Extend arms holding weight above face. BREATHE IN.*

4   *BREATHING OUT,*
      slowly takes the arms over and behind your head, holding the weight lengthways with both hands, pointing to the floor.

5   *Hold for a count of 3,*
      feeling a wonderful stretch throughout the body.

6   *BREATHING IN, slowly raise arms back into*
      the starting position.

Repeat 10 times. This completes one set.

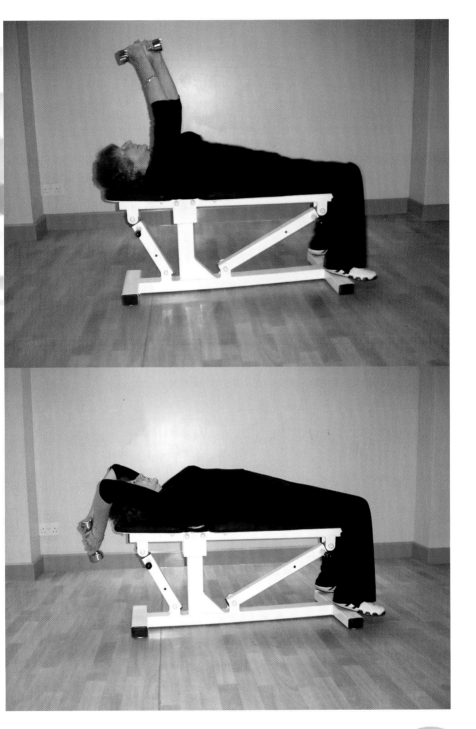

WORKING THE CHEST
INCLINED CHEST PRESS

Stretches and expands the chest, good for arms and shoulders. This exercise will also tone the bosom.

Do keep your arms bent as you lower them. Keeping them straight puts a strain on elbows and shoulders and makes the exercise much harder to do. You can improvise the equipment by using a chair for this exercise.

1   Prop up bench back support so that it is inclined. Sit down and lean back on to the support.

2   Tuck your chin in towards your chest, back should be in a normal posture, not arched or flattened.

3   Tighten the abdominals.

4   Hold the arms high over chest, straight but not locked. BREATHE IN.

5   BREATHING OUT slowly lower the arms sideways until approximately level with shoulders, maintaining a bend in elbows.

6   Slowly raise arms to starting position, keeping a wide distance between your arms until they join above your chest.

7   Repeat 10 times. This completes one set.

Aim to add another set as soon as possible.

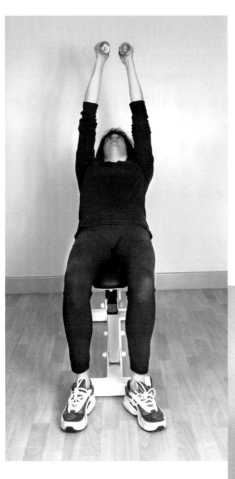

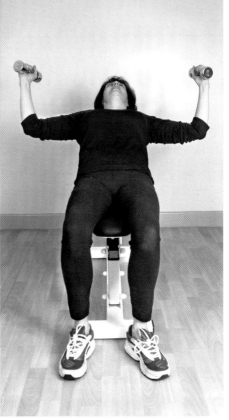

This exercise is also good for the shoulders and will help tone the arms

1   Stand upright, feet hip width apart. Do not lock the knees.
2   Hold light weights, (1kg may be enough to start).
3   Extend the arms to the front at shoulder height.
4   'Draw' small circles the size of saucers in the air.
5   Repeat 15 times. This completes one set.

Move on to heavier weights as you become stronger and when able, do another set.

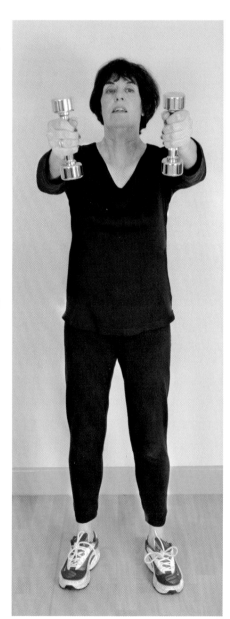

EXERCISE 10

WORKING THE SHOULDERS
THE SHRUG

Strengthens shoulders and upper back.

1 *Holding 1 kg or more weights, stand straight with knees loose, legs hip width apart, arms down by sides.*

2 *Let the arms down to their fullest extent, bend the knees slightly. BREATHE IN.*

3 *BREATHING OUT, shrug shoulders towards the ears, keeping the arms straight.*

4 *Repeat 15 times This completes one set.*

5 *Increase the weights as you gain strength.*

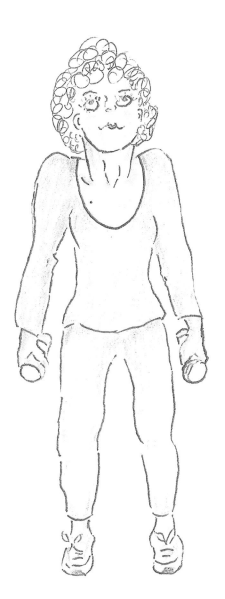

WORKING THE SHOULDERS
THE SHOULDER PRESS

Be careful if you have upper back or neck problems.
This will benefit the centre and tops of shoulder muscles, and it also works the upper back.

A chair can be used if you do not have a bench.

1   *Raise back of the bench to a sitting position*
     and raise seat slightly.

2   *Sit with back supported, abdomen pulled in towards your back.*
     There should be a slight gap between your back and the bench
     but do not let your back arch away from the bench.

3   *Hold weight with palms facing out at ear height. BREATHE IN.*

4   *BREATHING OUT - Raise arms above the head, as though you*
     were raising them around a barrel on your head.

5   *Bring weights together with arms high above head,*
     arms straight but not locked.

6   *Slowly lower to starting position.*

7   *Repeat 10 times. This completes one set.*

8   *Repeat the set.*

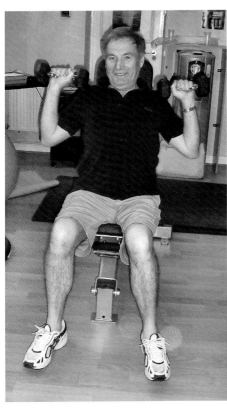

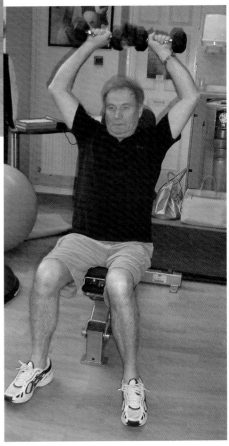

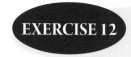

EXERCISE 12

WORKING THE SHOULDERS
REAR SHOULDER PULL

Many of the shoulder extensions do not exercise the back of the shoulder. This can result in poor posture, so do incorporate this exercise to keep everything nicely balanced.

If you have neck problems, it may be wise to give this a miss.

1   *Sit on the edge of the bench, holding a dumbbell in each hand, behind the ankles, palms facing inwards.*

2   *Lean forward from the hips so that your back is flat. Incline chin towards your chest and hold it in this position.*

3   *Stretch out the arms sideways keeping the elbows slightly bent.*

4   *Squeeze the shoulder blades together as you move the arms.*

5   *Slowly return to the starting position.*

6   *Repeat 10 times. This completes one set.*

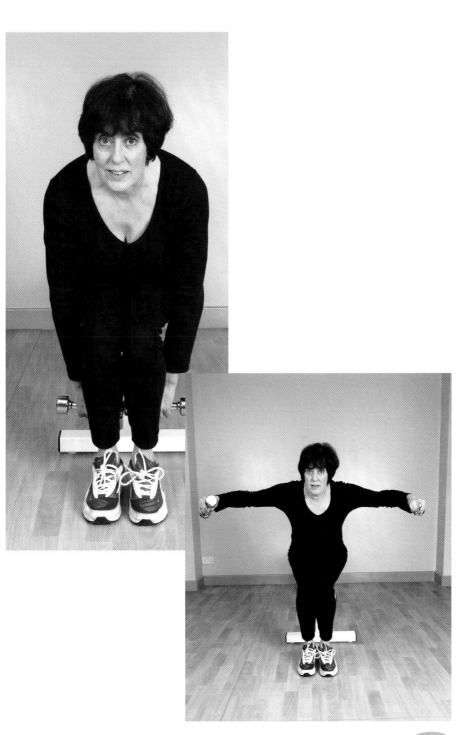

WORKING THE ARMS
THE BICEP CURL

1   *Sit on a bench or a chair with the legs slightly wider than hip width apart, lean forward slightly.*

2   *Hold a weight in the right hand; allow the right arm to hang straight down with the elbow against the inside of right knee.*

3   *Support your left side by placing your left wrist on the left knee.*

4   *BREATHE IN.*

5   *BREATHING OUT, bend the right arm, slowly raising the weight until almost at shoulder height.*

6   *Slowly return to starting position.*

7   *Make sure your movements are controlled.*

8   *Repeat on left side.*

9   *Repeat 10 times. This completes one set.*

10 *Repeat the set.*

In addition to strengthening the arms, this exercise will help to keep them toned and younger looking. It will enable you to bare your whole arms without cringing at the thought of exposing flab!

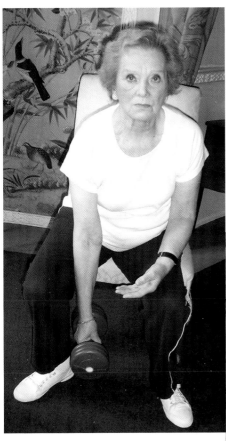

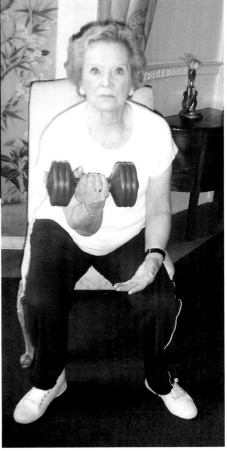

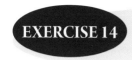

EXERCISE 14 *WORKING THE ABDOMINALS*
ABDOMINALS 1.

Abdominal strengthening, together with back strengthening exercises, will help give you strong core muscles, providing stability and good balance also, improving posture, breathing and digestion.

A gentle exercise, suitable for beginners to establish breathing and muscle control for all the abdominal exercises.

1   Lie on the floor with legs bent at the knees,
     chin lifted, but do not arch the neck.

2   Rest your hands alongside the tops of the thighs.

3   BREATHE IN, clench your abdominal muscles towards
     your spine and contract your pelvic muscles.

4   BREATHING OUT, slowly slide your hands up the thighs.

5   BREATHING IN, slowly lower to starting position.

6   Repeat 10 times. This completes one set.

7   Repeat the set.

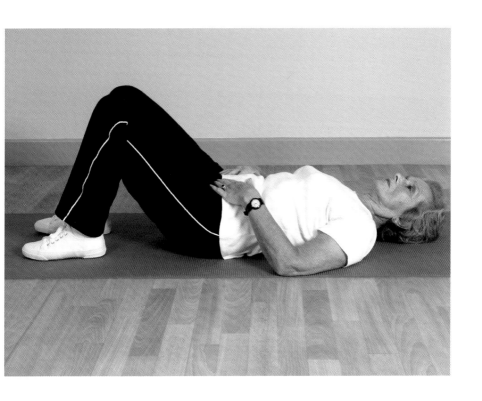

Stop and start again if you are not mastering the technique.
Work slowly and control your breathing so that you are breathing OUT as you lift, breathing in as you lower.

You should be clenching the muscles of the abdomen, as though they are trying to reach the spine and using those muscles to help you lift.

WORKING THE ABDOMINALS
THE ABDOMINAL CURL

This exercise may also help 'lift' that double chin.

1   *Lie on your back, with chin downwards but with some space between chin and chest; legs hip width apart.*

2   *Hands can either be stretched out in front over (although not touching) your knees, beside your ears or supporting your head, elbows held out.*

3   *Push your lower back into the floor, as though you are trying to make your navel touch your spine.*

4   *Clench your pelvic muscles (as for Pelvic Tilt).*

5   *BREATHE IN.*

6   *BREATHE OUT as you raise your shoulders about 2-3 inches from the floor in a curl, hold for a count of one.*

7   *Lower, pressing into the floor with your lower back all the time.*

8   *Repeat 10 times. This completes one set.*
   Add additional sets as you progress.

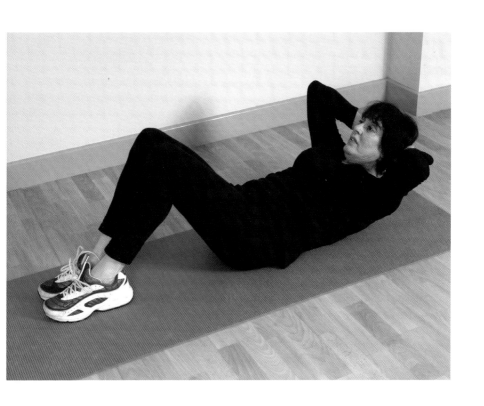

DO NOT LIFT WITH THE NECK. If you put strain on your neck you could achieve a very painful injury and it will not strengthen your abdomen.

Remember – it is the technique that is important, not the speed or the number of repeats.

EXERCISE 16 WORKING THE ABDOMINALS AND LOWER BACK - ABDOMINAL PLANK

Only progress to the Plank when you have gained strength in your lower back and abdominals, but beware if you have shoulder, back or arm problems, as this may not be for you. So give it a miss unless you are sure that you have no worries in these areas.

Tones the abs, strengthens the lower back and also works the shoulders and upper arms.

1   *Lie on the floor on your front, with forearms in front of your body, shoulder width   apart, feet together toes turned under, stomach touching the floor.*

2   *BREATHE IN.*

3   *BREATHING OUT, raise your body horizontally, keep it level and bearing your weight on the forearms and toes, keeping the head level and in line with the body.*

4   *Hold for as long as possible.*

5   *Breathing in, slowly lower to the ground.*

6   *Raise again and hold.*

As the exercise becomes easier, increase the holding time. It is quite good to time your holds so that you can chart your progress.

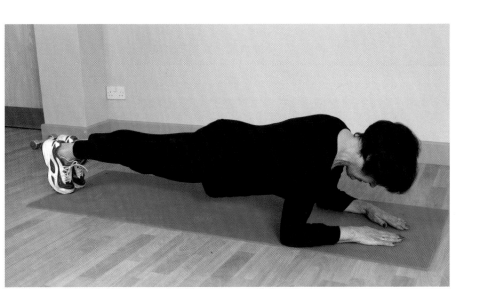

RECOGNISING A STROKE COULD SAVE A LIFE

These 4 small observations could save a life. Sometimes symptoms of a stroke are difficult to identify and the lack of awareness and consequent delay can be disastrous. A stroke victim may suffer severe brain damage when people nearby fail to recognise the symptoms. Doctors say a stroke can be recognised by asking 4 simple questions

1. *Ask the person to smile*
2. *Ask the person to speak a simple sentence.*
3. *Ask the person to raise both arms.*
4. *Ask the person to stick out their tongue.(Sign of a stroke is that the tongue is crooked – e.g. Going to one side or another.)*

*If the person has trouble with **ANY ONE** of these tasks describe the symptoms when you **CALL 999.***

Getting medical attention quickly is essential for stroke victims and may make the difference between recovery and permanent damage or death.

All the strengthening exercises for the lower body will also help enormously if you have poor circulation in the legs or 'puffy' ankles.

1   *Sit on the floor supported by the hands.*
       Legs straight out in front of you.

2   *Slowly raise right leg from the ground*
       as high as it is comfortable.

3   *Slowly bring it back towards the floor, but not touching the floor.*

4   *Raise again.*

5   *Repeat 10 times.*

6   *Repeat with the left leg. This completes one set.*

7   *Repeat the set.*

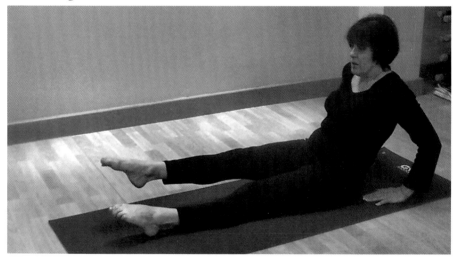

Many of the floor exercises can be slotted in to your day anytime you have a few minutes to spare.

EXERCISE 18

WORKING THE LEGS
LEG CIRCLES

1   Sit on the floor with legs straight in front of   you.

2   Raise one leg from the floor.

3   Circle the foot slowly with the heel raised from the floor.

4   Lower the foot to the floor.

5   Repeat 10 times.

6   Repeat with the other leg. This completes one set.

7   Repeat the set.

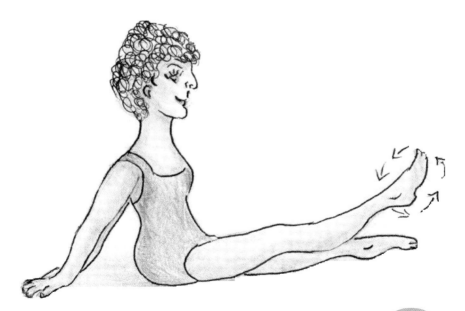

EXERCISE 19

WORKING THE LEGS
LEG CROSSOVER

1   Sit on the floor as before.
2   Lift the right leg slowly about 6" from the floor.
3   Cross over the left leg.
4   Slowly return to starting position.
5   Repeat 10 times.
6   Changeover to the right leg.
7   Repeat 10 times. This completes one set.
8   Repeat the set.

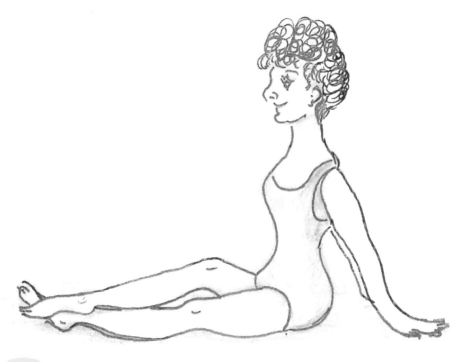

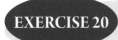

WORKING THE LEGS
KNEE TO CHEST

1   Sit on the floor with legs straight out in front of you,
      supported by your hands.

2   Raise one leg from the floor and then
      draw it into your chest.

3   Hold for a count of two and then straighten again.

4   Repeat 10 times.

5   Repeat with other leg.

This completes one set Repeat the set.

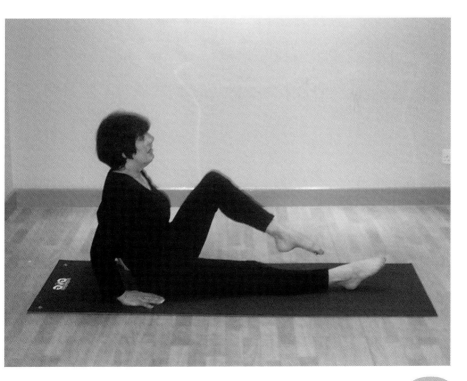

EXERCISE 21

HIP STRENGTHENER

The Hip Strengthener is very helpful if you have signs of early osteo-arthritis in the hips or stiffness in that area.

1   *Stand at a table or wall for support,
       with feet flat on the floor hip width apart.*

2   *Put all your body weight onto the left leg, weight can be
       increased by holding a hand weight in your left hand.*

3   *Raise the right foot off the ground (all your weight is supported
       by your left leg which should be straight, knee not locked).*

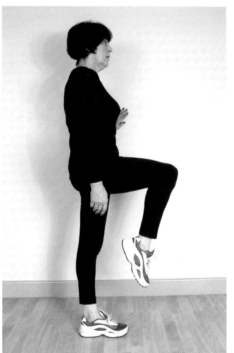

       Hold for 3 seconds.

4   *Lower to the ground.*

5   *Repeat 10 times.*

6   *Do not lock the knees.*

7   *Changeover to the other
       leg and changeover hand
       weight, if used.*

8   *Repeat 10 times.
       This completes one set.*

9   *Complete another set.*

This exercise will also help disperse cellulite from the thighs. Do this exercise, using a strong chair or stool, anytime you have a few spare minutes.

1   *Sit on the front edge of a chair with feet flat on the floor, arms crossed and keeping your back straight, lean forward a little.*

2   *Rise slowly to a standing position.*

3   *Pause and return to sitting position.*

4   *Repeat 10 times. This completes one set.*

5   *Repeat the set.*

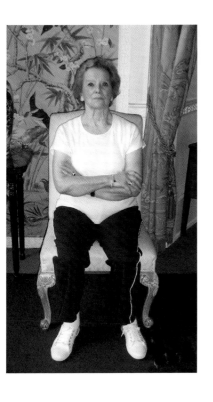
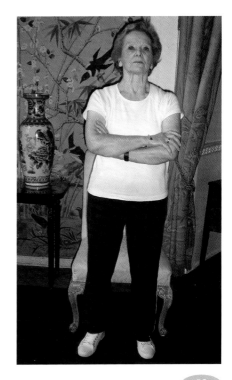

WORKING THE THIGHS
STRENGTHENS AND TONES

1   Stand with your head and back against a wall
     Position your feet 18 inches in front of you, hip width apart.

2   Slide your body down the wall until you are in a seated position.

3   Hold for a count of 10

4   Slowly slide your body back to the starting position.

5   Repeat once.

6   Relax.

Over a period increase the amount of holding time

Increase repeats to 4 when possible.

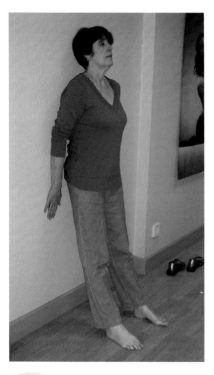 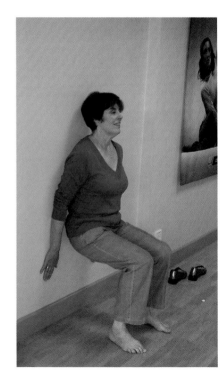

EXERCISE 24 — *WORKING THE LOWER LEGS - LOWER LEG STRETCHER*

1   *This exercise will stretch muscles and help to increase blood flow in the feet and lower legs.*
The bottom step of the stairs is ideal for this exercise,
you do not need to wear trainers and will probably be more stable on carpet with bare feet.

2   **Stand on a step, or the bottom step of a staircase with the toes and balls of the feet on the step, heels hanging in space.**

3   **Support yourself with one hand on a rail or wall.**

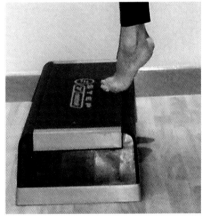

4   **Rise up as high as possible on to toes and hold for a count of three.**

5   **Slowly lower, dropping the heels down until they are below the level of the step.**

6   **Repeat 10 times. This completes one set.**

7   **Repeat the set.**

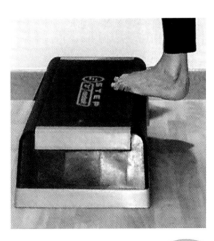

When you become proficient at this exercise, make it harder by hooking one foot behind the opposite calf, so that all your weight is borne by one foot.

WORKING THE ANKLES
ANKLE STRENGTHENER

1   Stand about 12 inches from a wall.

2   Feet should be shoulder width apart.

3   Rest hands lightly on the wall just to maintain your balance.

4   Slowly rise up as high as possible on the balls of your feet.

5   Hold for three seconds.

6   Lower to starting position.

7   Repeat 10 times, rest. This completes one set.

8   Repeat the set.

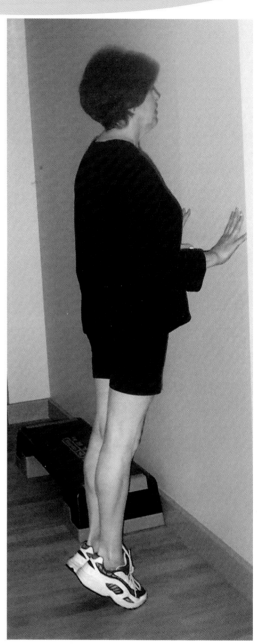

CONGRATULATIONS

You have completed the programme

Now, another whole body stretch to relax the muscles and cool down:-

Stand with left hand holding a bar (a door frame will do the job too), lean away from the frame, stretching the whole body from the feet upwards. Turn the body slightly to the right and stretch the right arm out away from the body.

Repeat three times and then changeover to the right side.

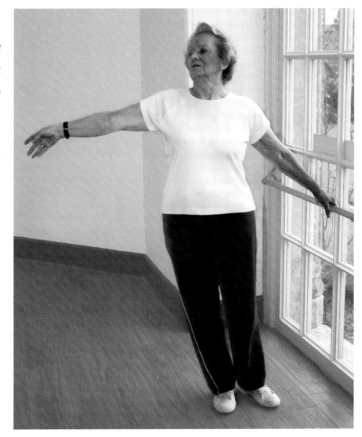

We have included these water based exercises as a change from your weights at home or the gym, they are not meant as an alternative, but perhaps to include once each week.

Walking in water may be advocated by your medical advisor following knee or hip replacement surgery. It enables you to exercise without placing pressure upon joints.

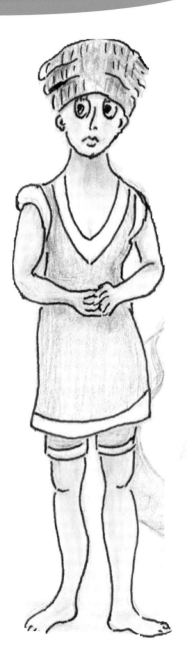

WARMING UP

Spend 10-20 minutes warming up by walking in the pool at chest depth, not easy but you will improve with each session. Try to keep your heels down as walking on your toes will give you aching calf muscles the next day.

Swimming of course will warm your blood prior to strength exercising and is an excellent exercise, but it is NOT WEIGHT BEARING and will not aid bone density.

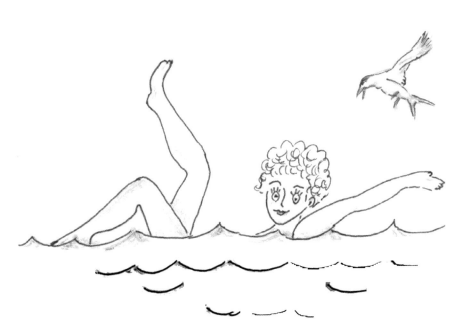

EXERCISE 26

**EXERCISING THE ARMS,
SHOULDERS AND BACK**

1   Stand facing the edge of the pool; place your hands on the edge.

2   Bending your knees, lower yourself down into the water.

3   Inhale

4   Exhaling, lever yourself up as far as you can, straightening
     the legs but keeping relaxed

5   Lift up out of the water, bearing your weight on your hands
     and arms, keeping your back straight.

6   Hold for a count of 1-3

7   Return to the starting position

8   Repeat, aiming to raise repeats to 10 as you gain in strength

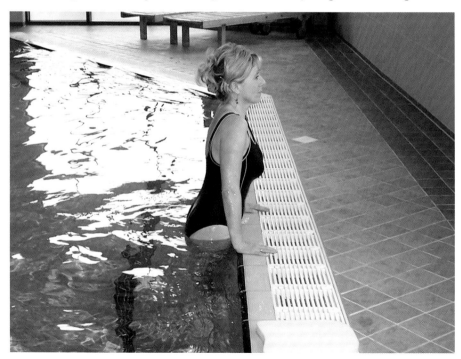

result
result
result

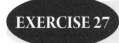

STRENGTHENING
THE ARMS AND SHOULDERS

1   *Using water dumbbells,*
    stand with your hands in front of you, facing downwards,
    holding the dumbbells on the surface of the water, arms bent
2   *Inhale .*
3   *Exhaling, push the dumbbells down in front of you*
    until your hands are level with your thighs and are straight,
    do not lock the elbows.
4   *Slowly raise the dumbbells to the surface again.*
5   *Repeat 10 times, building up repeats as you gain strength.*

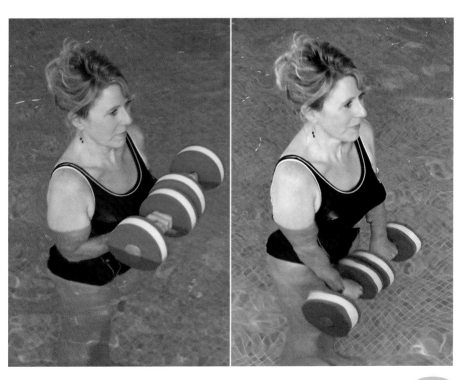

(Much harder than the previous exercise but will work wonders for your upper arms, keeping them strong and looking good (think of those short sleeves in summer). Excellent also for preventing batwings:-

1   *Standing holding the dumbbells on the surface of the water, hands facing UPWARDS.*

2   *Inhale.*

3   *Exhaling, slowly push down in front of your body until your arms are fully extended.*

4   *Release and raise slowly to the surface again.*

5   *Repeat 10 times, gradually increasing repeats as you gain strength.*

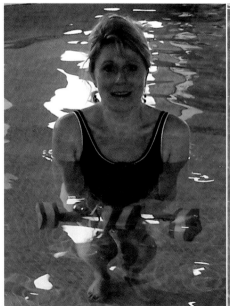
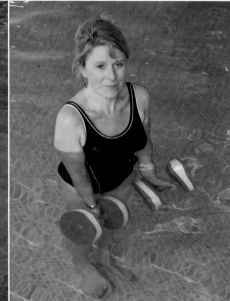

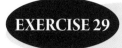

EXERCISING THE CHEST

1   Stand in water up to chest level.
2   Stretch out hands to each side with palms facing forward.
3   Inhale.
4   Exhaling, turn the hands and sweep them backwards
      as far as possible.
5   Turn the hands to palms facing forwards again and
      bring them slowly in front of you.
6   Return to starting position.
7   Repeat 10 times.

To make this harder, try holding a water dumbbell in each hand.

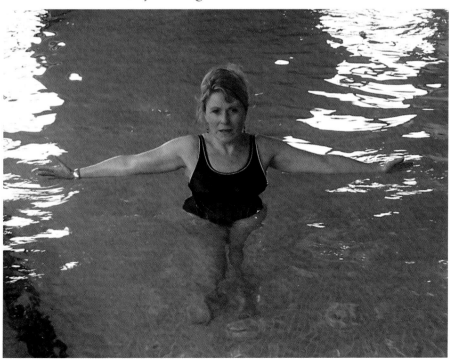

1   *Using the edge of the pool to hold.*

2   *Face towards the pool, back to the edge, upright in the water and bring your legs at right angles to your trunk*
(into a seated position but with the legs straight out in front).

3   *Form a V shape with your legs.*

4   *Hold for 10-20 seconds.*

5   *Slowly bring the legs back together and lower.*

6   *Repeat 10 times, increasing repeats as you gain strength. Breathe slowly and evenly throughout this exercise.*

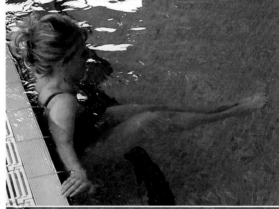

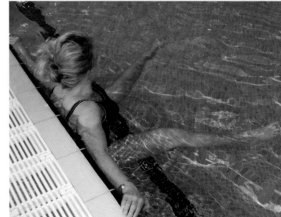

EXERCISING THE ABDOMINALS

1 Stand in the water placing
   your elbows or hands,
   whichever suits you, on
   the edge of the pool
   for support.
2 Stretch the legs
   straight in front of you.
3 Inhale.
4 Exhaling, bring your
   knees up to your
   chest and hold
   for 10 seconds.
5 Straighten to the front and
   then lower again.
   Repeat 10 times
   extending as you progress.

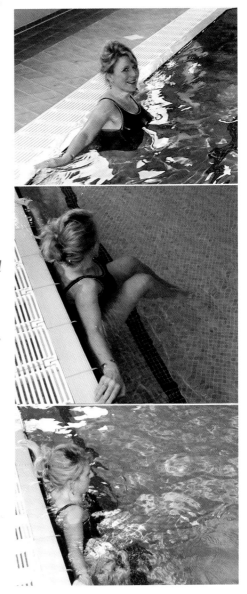

1   Using a float or dumbbells for support,
     pedal the legs in the water
     (as though you are riding a bike).
2   Work both forwards and backwards.
3   Do this for 10 minutes or work up to 10 minutes over a period.

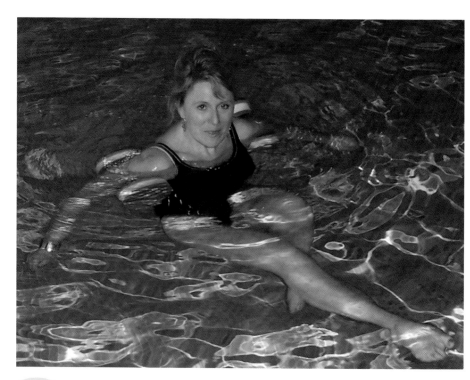

ANOTHER ONE FOR HIPS AND LEGS

Using a float, lie face down on the water and
scissor your legs backwards.
Can also be performed holding on to the side of the pool.
The scissoring movement will work the hips, tone the backside and work
the legs.
Do this for as long as you can.

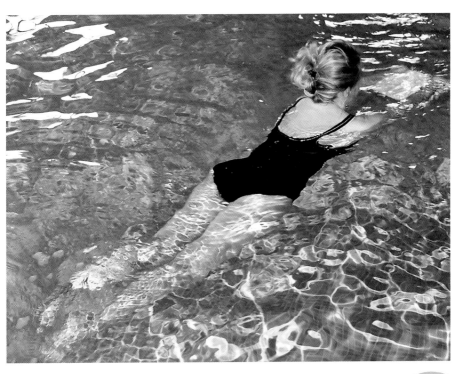

EXERCISE 34 — *EXERCISING THE FEET AND ANKLES*

Supporting yourself on the edge of the pool, or on a bar
(not putting weight onto your hands and arms).

1   *Rise up on to your toes and hold for a count of 3.*

2   *Slowly lower heels to the ground.*

3   *Repeat 10 times.*

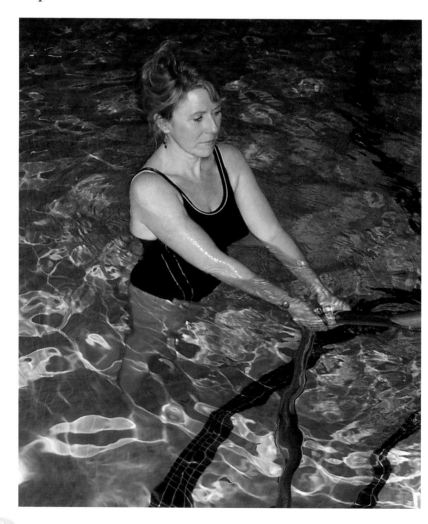

EXERCISING FROM A CHAIR

If you are unable to stand or have difficulty in balancing, try exercising from a sitting position.

If you are unfit, a stranger to exercise, are taking medication or suffering from any medical condition seek your doctor's advice before taking any exercise or making a change in your lifestyle.

Also, when you start exercising under any of these circumstances, it is best to have someone else present to help if needed.

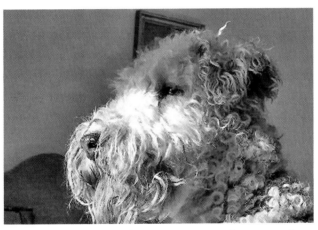

If you are lacking incentive to take exercise, get a dog, Your dog will have to be walked each day which will get you out too, and there is nothing like the boundless loyalty, devotion and companionship of a dog to give you peace and tranquility and reduce the stress in your life. The Dog's Trust always has a good selection of dogs of all ages looking for a new home, and it may be a good idea to select an older dog if you are not in the first flush of youth. If owning a dog is impossible, then offer to exercise a friend's dog. You will definitely gain two new best friends!

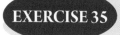

IMPROVING
THE CIRCULATION

1   *Sit back in your chair, take two deep breaths.*

2   *Rest feet on your heels and spread out toes,*
        at the same time spreading out the fingers in front of you.

3   *Clench the hands, curl the toes then release*

4   *Repeat as many times as you can manage,*
        ideally commencing at 5 repeats and increasing to 20.

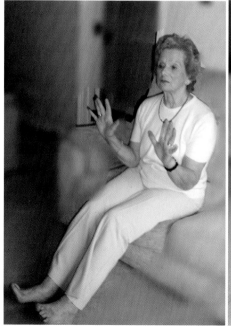
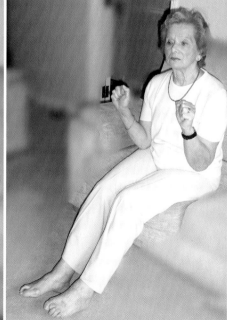